▶ ▶ ▶ Keys to Winning Physician Support

A Guide for Executives and Managers

by Richard E. Thompson, MD

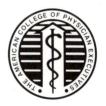

The American College of Physician Executives

Two Urban Centre, Suite 200
4890 West Kennedy Boulevard
Tampa, Florida 33609
(813) 287-2000

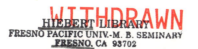

For the Busy Executive

 Throughout this book, key points are summarized in boxes such as this one.

This book is designed for the busy executive to use in two ways:

- Read it (or at least scan the executive summary boxes).

- Discuss key points in executive/physician meetings, study groups, and retreats.

A Brief Glossary

The following are context definitions of a few key words and phrases used
in this book:

Physician—An MD or DO whose training is primarily clinical, and whose
major activity is providing direct patient care.

Executive—A person whose training is primarily in business, finance,
managing data and people, and establishing working systems. Executives
in an organization are given, by the owners and through a governing body,
responsibility and limited authority to carry out (execute) the principles,
policies, goals, plans, and objectives of the organization.

Physician executive—An individual who, in whatever sequence, has
acquired both clinical and executive expertise and whose primary activities
as an executive include interacting with both physicians and executives.

Clinical Expertise—A body of knowledge and skills dealing with the
anatomy and physiology of the human body and with diagnosis and
treatment of illness and injury.

Practice—As applied to physicians in this book, "practice" does *not* refer to
traditional "private practice." Examples of practicing physicians include a
hospital–based anesthesiologist, an internist in "private practice," a general
surgeon employed by or contracting with a managed care organization, a
family physician in a large multispecialty clinic, and a skilled subspecialist
on the faculty of a medical university.

System—The effort of several individuals, often with disparate training
and experience, exercised in concert, to successfully accomplish a stated
task.

Foreword

The American College of Physician Executives commissioned this book primarily for use by its members. But this book can be useful to any executive who works in the same environment with actively practicing physicians.

The book emphasizes the evolving role of the Vice President, Medical Services (Medical Director), in settings that include a traditionally organized medical staff. But many points in this book are applicable to any setting in which executives and physicians are co–workers.

Introduction

I had experience working with [hospital management] students...who never had exposure to a nurse or a doctor. The one opportunity they had to understand what a doctor or a nurse does (their training) had been blown. They need to understand what makes a nurse and doctor work, what are their value judgments, and how to get them to be a part of the team.—H. Robert Cathcart, CEO, Pennsylvania Hospital, Philadelphia, Pa.

The success of any health care executive depends, in part, on understanding the value judgments and informal power of even a small group of physicians, who may not even be major players in the organization. ◀◀◀

Not all health care executive training programs stress the importance of learning and dealing with the unique characteristics of physician behavior (see Chapter 1). Ironically, even *physician* executives may forget, or disregard, the impact of physicians' value judgments on success or failure of the organization's plans.

Working together, the executive team and physician leaders who are primarily clinical practitioners can design and implement strategies that reasonable "follower" physicians will welcome and embrace. Simultaneously, the informal power of ever–present, highly visible, emotional, "loyal opposition" physicians will be lessened.

Physician executives are uniquely positioned to lead the development of mutually beneficial working relationships with a wider network of physicians. This is a critically important priority. One first step toward the promise of tomorrow is putting aside yesterday's notion that executive–physician conflict is inevitable.

About the Author

Richard E. Thompson, MD, is a member of the American College of Physician Executives and a frequent member of the faculty of the Congress on Administration of the American College of Healthcare Executives. He is a graduate of Vanderbilt University and Washington University School of Medicine (MD, cum laude, AOA, 1959.) Once in private pediatric practice, then hospital–based chair of pediatrics in a 500–bed medical center and assistant professor of pediatrics in the Emory University School of Medicine, he was a member of the staff of the Joint Commission on Accreditation of Hospitals (now the Joint Commission on Accreditation of Healthcare Organizations)(1974–75) and vice president of the Illinois Hospital Research and Education Foundation (1975–79). Since 1979, Dr. Thompson has been president of Thompson, Mohr, and Associates, Inc., P.O. Box 1497, Dunedin, Florida 34697-1497, 813/937-0170.

Other books by Dr. Thompson include *The Medical Staff Leader's Complete Practical Guidebook, Next Steps in Implementing Quality Improvement, The CEO's and Board Member's Guide to Medical Staff Structure and Responsibilities,* and *Keys to Winning Physician Support.*

Dr. Thompson is a speaker, consultant, author, and innovator who has been introduced as equally trusted in executive offices, the board room, and the doctors' lounge.

Table of Contents

Part I—The Executive/Physician Interface

Part II—Critical Guidelines

Part III—Some Practical Examples

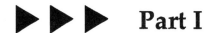 Part I

The Executive/Physician Interface

Chapter 1

Conflicting Characteristics of Executives and Physicians

The [presence of] the professions means that the modern large–scale organization has been heavily infiltrated by people who have an entirely different concept of what organization is about....In effect, these people are 'outsiders' working within the system.

At the same time, the term "profession" is itself taking on new meaning....People increasingly find that the novel problems thrust at them can be solved only by reaching beyond narrow disciplines.—John Gardner, cited in *Future Shock* by Alvin Toffler, Bantam Books, 1971, p. 147.

Until recently, with a few exceptions, the term "physician executive" was an oxymoron.

The conflicting nature of the basic characteristics of business executives and of physicians are shown in the table on page 2. Executives relate to other individuals and groups with an understanding of systems and common goals. On the other hand, physicians are usually individualists. The physician's main relationship to other individuals and groups is primarily a herd behavior, grouping with others of the same kind, with the goal of protecting the individuality of each member of the herd. This behavior could also be likened to settlers moving West in a wagon train, each family fiercely independent, yet together circling the wagons when necessary to fight off threats to the different goals pursued by each.

These conflicting characteristics make it difficult for executives and practicing physicians to appreciate each other's worlds. In fact, two common causes of frustration, for both executives and physicians, are:

1

Table 1

Characteristics of Executives and Physicians

Executives	Practicing Physicians
Trained in and concerned with financial matters (budget, acquisitions, marketing, etc.), group process, personnel management, legalities, external regulations.	Trained in and concerned with disorders in anatomy and/or physiology of the human body; diagnosis and treatment of illness and injury, in a chosen limited clinical field.
Understands that executive privilege is limited by higher authority... governing body policies and organizational goals.	Often appears to believe that there is no higher authority, even, in some instances, The Law.
Data–oriented. Is justifiably concerned with what happens to groups of patients...impact of decisions and actions on the goals of the organization for which the executive has been made responsible by the governing body.	Case–oriented. Is justifiably concerned with what happens to an individual... impact of decisions and actions on the welfare of patients for which the practitioner is responsible. May not appreciate the value of accumulating and using data, over time.
Responsible for implementing change.	Many with Gloria Patri Mentality. As it was in the beginning, is now and ever shall be.
Must manage to stay within budget, or control costs to maximize profit, depending on the specific healthcare setting.	May have little experience with planning and limiting expenditures, because of (up to now) large amounts of expendable income.
Delegates responsibilities; go do it and report back.	Fears being "disenfranchised;" don't do anything without asking me first.
Expects to be evaluated.	May view suggestions about how to practice medicine, or even about other matters, as "interference" with a physician's "prerogative."
Allegiance is primarily to the organization employing the executive at the moment; secondarily to others in the same field through colleges and associations.	Allegiance is primarily to other practitioners, through practice arrangements, specialty societies, and local, state, and national associations.

- Many physicians still do not understand the health care center as an organization. So when physicians glibly agree to abide by organizational rules, such as medical staff bylaws, they may not really understand that they are agreeing to recognize the authority of the Medical Executive Committee, clinical department chairs, the vice president of medical services, the governing body, and the chief executive officer. (Of course, it is easier for everyone, including physicians, when the relative responsibility and authority of these individuals and groups is carefully clarified).

- At the same time, people with business training tend to take approaches to physicians that reflect the world of business, but not the world of clinical practice.

In the absence of formal cross–training in graduate schools (a deficiency that should be remedied), balanced understanding comes slowly. And in the absence of understanding, mistaken judgments about each other may be made. For example, some physicians tend to blame "administration" when traditional expectations are disappointed. But it is not the fault of health care executives that physicians no longer enjoy autonomy and nearly unlimited income. In fact, executives are as frustrated as physicians by decreased revenue, a litigious environment, political chicanery, and increased central government control.

In the absence of cross–training, executives emphasizing similarities between the health care business and other businesses may tend to overlook important differences. And one big difference is the undeniable presence of physician factors in the health care equation.

But a significant number of physicians and executives now understand that one's success depends on the other. The problem is that neither group quite knows how to take the first step toward the other. Thus the new breed of physician executive joins a cast of players eager to take advantage of mutually productive efforts, but unsure about how to proceed.

One of the first steps is to identify, and define the relationship between, two different kinds of physician leader:

- Physician leaders, who are primarily practitioners, such as chairs of clinical departments of a medical staff, multispecialty clinic, or managed care physician group.

- Physician executives, who understand clinician's concerns but whose executive skills and position of authority make them valuable, full–time members of the inner circle of senior executives.

A major role of the second group can be to orient and guide individuals in the first group.

One thorny problem will probably be with us for some time. Some physicians are reluctant to accept leadership from a full–time physician executive. A few may persist in believing that such an individual has "gone over to the other side."

Even as the physician executive provides a physician voice in high level decision–making circles, some physicians may distrust a fair, objective physician executive simply because he or she *is* a member of the inner circle of senior executives.

The number of such physicians is smaller than it was a few years ago, but even a small number of such physicians can create difficulties for the physician executive. Physician executives should be less concerned with the number of such individuals than with the potential impact of even a few.

An MD or DO degree does not automatically make a physician executive acceptable to physicians. It is important to spend time listening to, taking reasonable suggestions from, and gradually gaining the support of reasonable practitioners.

Chapter 2

The Importance of Physician Support

The executive/management staff must care what physicians think about planned projects. The alternative is risking delay or even failure, in spite of sound financial and legal planning.

The importance of physician support is illustrated by the following true–life examples encountered by the author in his consulting practice:

- "Our merger isn't working out exactly as we planned, because primary care physicians continue their traditional referral patterns. We assumed that primary care physicians would start referring to specialists in the hospital with which we merged. We're way short of revenue projections, based on assumptions about admission and referral patterns of our docs. Where did we go wrong?" (A word to the wise: Some physicians react negatively to being referred to as "docs.")

- "A few physicians are killing us, economically, by overutilizing diagnostic services and needlessly extending hospital stays. Attempts to feed this information back as part of routine reappointment almost caused a 'palace revolt.' Some of the docs called it 'economic credentialing.' Why don't they trust us?"

- "Control of physicians is supposed to be through the organized medical staff. But 90 percent of our physicians are apathetic; they don't participate in the organization, except to send in a "No" on a mail ballot. Medical staff reorganization is a high priority with us, but not with them. Why can't they see they're making us all vulnerable by refusing to change?"

- "Some specialists on our staff are battling over certain privileges, such as laparoscopy and use of special care units. Physicians on the Credentials Committee and Medical Executive Committee are making some credentialing recommendations that may get us in serious legal difficulty. How would you handle that?"

- "We joint ventured a diagnostic service with a few of our physicians. It looked like a good idea on paper. But we angered a majority of our physicians, who are now boycotting the venture, which is losing money. The outsider physicians are telling their board member friends that this is just one example of 'poor management decisions.' I could even lose my job over this."

- "Our medical center did beautifully in the Joint Commission survey, except for some Type I recommendations (reportable to HCFA if we do not get them removed), all related to ineffective medical staff functions. The thousands of dollars and hours of staff time spent to relieve those Type I recommendations relates directly back to refusal of three clinical department chairs to do their jobs. How should our physician leaders be oriented?"

- "We are well into implementing total quality management, focusing on the integrity of systems. Now, we are discovering that industrial TQM models don't always deal with the reality of relatively uncontrolled physician judgments, which continue to be necessary because care must be individualized to some extent. How do you incorporate the physician factor into a total quality management process?"

- "How do we reconcile the hospital's interest in new outpatient services and wellness programs with physicians' interest in hospitalizing people, ordering drugs, and doing surgery?"

- "We would have a medical director/vice president of medical services by now, except that a few physicians equate establishing this position with 'surrendering more control over doctors to the hospital.' What would you do?"

- "Our physicians really should be our marketing program. But we understand from employees, who learn it from friends, that some of our physicians are bad–mouthing the hospital to patients in their offices. Our market share is down. We don't know if that's a factor or not. How should we find out?"

Executives must respond to board members' increased interest in medical staff matters. Sometimes the board is concerned about occupancy rates and profit. Sometimes there is a genuine altruistic interest in dependable health care services for the community, beginning with consistent performance by the health care center's physicians. And sometimes, a troublesome, costly lawsuit has exposed shortcomings in the health care center's credentialing and "peer review" mechanisms.

Physician support can also be important to the career goals of the health care executive. At least anecdotally, it is hard to deny a relationship between executive turnover and medical staff unrest. At least to some extent, physician executives may share this occupational hazard with nonphysician executives! The bottom line is that divisive behavior erodes trust, costs money, and increases *everybody's* vulnerability.

Viewed in terms of productivity, time spent winning physician support is productive time indeed.

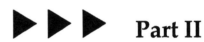 Part II

Critical Guidelines

Chapter 3

Defining the Role of Each Physician at the Health Care Center

Originally, physicians had only one role in a hospital setting. Each ◀◀◀ physician hospitalized, diagnosed, and treated/operated on patients from his own private practice. In contrast, physicians choose from a variety of available roles in today's health care organization (see figure on page 12).

Plaques and portraits in hospital lobbies reflect a Golden Age, when hospitals were established by forward–looking physician–philanthropist collaborators. The physician wanted hospital services for his patients; the philanthropic family wanted its community to have the very best in medical care. The resulting facility was often referred to as "the Doctor's Workshop."

In that old model, roles and relationships were simple. The physician ran his private office, hospitalizing and operating on patients solely at his discretion. The philanthropist chaired a board of trustees, the members of which were expected to contribute financially to the hospital. An administrator (once called a superintendent) ran the business side of the hospital, and direct patient care services were coordinated by a "chief nurse."

Many contemporary physicians grew up, professionally speaking, with this image of what a hospital should be. The author is a case in point. When Charles C. Dimmitt founded Dimmitt Memorial Hospital in Humansville, Missouri, in the 1930s, he appointed his young executive assistant, Guy Thompson (the author's father) as superintendent. Dad's correspondence indicates that he was chief executive officer, chief finance officer, public relations director, accountant, tax advisor, planner, and board secretary, plus personal confidant to Mr. Dimmitt, who was, of course, chairman of the

Generic Organizational Functions

Worker Function

Technical skills

Best knowledge of product design, production problems, and public reaction

Frontline interaction with people served by the organization

Motivated by adequate salary and benefits, but also by pride in one's contribution; satisfaction in a job well done

Director/Manager Function

Responsible for dependable performance of one component of the organization/business

Systems

Workers

Documentation

Evaluation

Executive Function

Execute

Assist, guide, support

Supervise

External relationships

On-site governing body authority

Coordinate

Governance Function

Ownership

Fiduciary accountability

Policies, corporate culture

Dispute resolution

Political action

Community visibility

People Served by the Business/Organization Expecting a Dependable Service or Product

board. (There were no such duties as marketing, utilization management, risk management, or accreditation/regulation.)

But the real decision–maker at Dimmitt Memorial Hospital was A.J. Stufflebaum, MD, the community's predominant physician. Mr. Thompson was frequently instructed by Mr. Dimmitt to "check with Dr. Stufflebaum." Perhaps that experience drove my father's desire that I become an MD. His experience taught him that, in those days, the physicians dealt the cards and named the game. Perhaps the only reason Dad became an attorney rather than a doctor was that he fainted at the sight of blood.

Disappointed expectations of physicians who feel that the rule still should be "check with Dr. Stufflebaum" and who believe that a medical center is still "the doctor's workshop" offer a major challenge to executives seeking to win physician support while at the same time exercising authority granted to the executive staff by the governing body.

The figure on the left illustrates the roles available in any organization. Physicians, by their actions, select for themselves the role(s) they wish to play at the health care center. The problem is that many physicians are unaware of the nature or meaning of their choices, because organizational theory is not part of medical training.

The executive staff and physician leaders may wish to use the figure on the left as a focus for discussion with physicians, to clarify roles available in today's health care organization.

Worker

Some physicians just want to be left alone. These individuals are interested in a relatively narrow aspect of health care (prescribing drugs, performing surgery, and/or performing invasive diagnostic procedures). These individuals are apathetic about organizational matters, attend meetings only to meet minimum requirements, and don't care to accept positions of organizational leadership. In addition, some of these individuals may resent assignments made by staff leaders, such as serving for a month or two as clinical analyst of physician performance data or being included on an emergency services call roster. But (make no mistake about it), some of these individuals are among the health care center's best clinicians and may care for families of other physicians, the executive staff, and board members.

Bylaws and rules can, and should, be crafted so that the worker option is available to physicians. But, in fairness, the ramification of this choice must be made clear. A physician who accepts the role of worker must accept the authority of others in the organization and is not entitled to go around acting as if he owns the place (see **Owner**, page 16).

Manager/Director

 The trend in traditional medical staff organizations is *from* government by committee *to* day–to–day management by responsible individuals, such as clinical department chairs.

A physician who chooses to accept the role of clinical department chair (service chief) must understand that organizational skills, as well as clinical skills, are now required. Language such as the following is now common in medical staff bylaws:

"In selecting department chairs, the staff shall consider interest, availability, organizational skills, written and oral communication skills, and reputation for objectivity and fairness necessary to fulfill assigned duties and to ensure appropriate physician participation in health care center affairs."

It is now critically important to address issues of selection, terms, orientation, and evaluation of clinical department chairs. It is also important to consider paying these leaders, such as from a joint physician/health care center "leadership payment fund."[1]

A medical director/vice president for medical services can "coach" clinical department chairs, who must perform organizational functions but who are still primarily clinicians.

Executive

Executives are responsible for carrying out plans and policies, and fulfilling stated objectives, of an organization. The chief executive officer is selected by the governing body, members of which govern the organization on behalf of the owners.

There is also an executive function in the traditional organized medical staff. The organized medical staff is one of the few organizations (if not the only organization) in which the executive function is assigned to a committee rather than to an individual. In this traditional model, the medical executive committee (MEC) is the highest physician authority but is subject to the authority of the governing body. Ordinarily, members of the MEC have little or no experience as executives.

Current trends suggest that the traditional executive committee model will give way to a vice president of medical services plus an advisory group or cabinet of five to seven physicians who are well–respected by physicians, board members, and the organization's executive staff (see Chapter 13).

Governor

Including physicians on the governing body is now the norm. And there is even variation in physician member roles on the board. That is, some physicians are expected to speak on behalf of the health care center's physicians, and some are expected to have a broader perspective.

There has never been any confusion about whether the board or the medical staff has the final say. The board has that authority and responsibility, because they represent the owners of the health care center. In 1917, the first description of an organized medical staff stated that "rules and regulations (are) subject to approval of the board."[2]

But confusion arose, because boards of trustees (directors) did not start exercising their authority, with regard to physician–related issues, until the 1970s. Prior to that time, board composition was not an issue to physicians, because boards ordinarily accepted ("rubber–stamped") physician suggestions and decisions. Not any more.

In the early 1970s, first efforts by physicians to obtain board seats were met with rejection, because nonphysician board members feared that some physicians might use seats on the board to pursue their own interests, rather than the interests of the community and the health care center. Yet, boards recognized the need for input from knowledgeable, reasonable physicians. The dilemma was resolved by placing one or two physicians on the board and carefully orienting these individuals to their responsibilities. That is, they were (and are) to have a broad perspective, not pursue physician interests.

Some physicians cried foul, believing (justifiably, to some extent) that physician interests *should* be included in discussions and decisions of the board. So, by 1990, elected officials of the medical staff (staff president, president-elect, and/or immediate past president) were added to the board. These individuals are expected to have a broad perspective, but also to speak for the health care center's medical staff (not for any individual, practice group, or specialty self–interest).

Trends suggest that health care center boards may become smaller and equally representative of ownership, executive expertise, and professional/ clinical expertise. (Physicians should note that nurses and others with "professional/clinical expertise" will also be eligible for those seats).

Owner

A physician is only entitled to act as if he owns the place if he really *does* own the place. For example, a group of physician investors may start or buy a hospital and establish a physician–majority board. Or a hospital in economic difficulty may save itself by jointly owning buildings and other health care center assets with physician investors. In that case, the executive staff and board have decided, whether consciously or not, to share power with physician investors.

Focusing on the concept of ownership, and on the necessity to choose or be assigned a role within the organization, is a valid way to define the relationship of individual physicians to this health care organization.

A physician may, of course, have more than one role. For example, a clinical department chair (director/manager function) is ordinarily also an active clinical practitioner (worker function). The key is to help physicians know which hat they are wearing in specific situations. A surgeon operating on his own patient, or participating as a consultant or assistant at the request of an attending physician, is wearing the hat of worker. The same surgeon who observes an operation for the purpose of "proctoring" a new staff member is wearing the hat of organizational leader, with a different responsibility and different legal liability. But the difference is not automatically clear to the surgeon, because the anatomical field laid open on the operating table looks the same in both instances.

A surgeon struggling to view operations on patients in the context of organizational principles is an image that graphically illustrates the challenge to executives working with physicians.

References

1. Thompson, R. "Paying Medical Staff Leaders for Organizational Responsibilities: The Time Has Come." *The Medical Staff Counselor*, 5(2):51-8, Spring 1991.

2. *The Minimum Standard*. Chicago, Ill.: American College of Surgeons, 1919.

Chapter 4

Ten Common Mistakes Executives Make When Dealing with Physicians

Mistake 1—Executives look for "an approach" to the medical staff.

There is no such thing as a single successful approach to a group of physicians. Rather, any approach must reflect the unique characteristics of several subgroups. The successful executive recognizes, and deals differently, with:

- **Dr. Wonderful:** Clinical skills, cooperative attitude, sense of responsibility, and sense of humor make this physician a delightful working companion.

- **Dr. Today:** Reluctant to change (who isn't?), but willing to change if convinced by persuasive arguments that change is necessary.

- **Dr. Yesterday:** Has the Gloria Patri mentality—"As it was in the beginning, is now and ever shall be."

- **Dr. Tomorrow:** The physician's vision matches that of health care executives.

- **Dr. Scientific:** This committed subspecialist seeks only to advance the art of medicine.

- **Dr. Entrepreneur:** May be a subspecialist in a highly technical, high revenue–producing clinical area; may be an economic partner of the health care organization in some joint venture.

- **Dr. Trouble:** Usually has excellent oratorical skills. Urges colleagues not to "collaborate with the enemy" (health care executives; insurance companies; attorneys; and, in some instances, just about everybody with whom this person comes in contact).

- **The Warrior:** May be working on, or have obtained, a law degree. Begins most sentences, "On the advice of legal counsel...." Handle with care.

Mistake 2—Cronyism.

Favoritism usually generates a significant number of disenchanted outsiders. It's fine to play golf with a few physicians whose frequent admissions or high–tech activities provide a major portion of "income from operations." But, don't ignore even occasional admitters who might negatively influence a large number of staff members.

Don't focus only on elected physician leaders and heavy admitters. Who are the *Informal* physician leaders, and what are they saying in the doctor's lounge?

Mistake 3—Fear of physicians.

Job security is a strong motivation, and executive turnover is sometimes related to medical staff unrest. Still, it is a mistake for executives to base their actions on fear of physicians. Reasonable physicians (even the blustery intimidators) respect, and eventually come to support, a person who chooses his or her ground carefully and then effectively defends it.

Fear is a mistake for several reasons. First, the executive staff cannot relinquish authority and control to a physician group. Also, the executive staff can be made to appear secretive and Machiavellian if its members fear sharing information with physicians. And trying too hard to please the most vocal physicians can actually result in losing support of a majority of the physician group. Finally, that old adage, "The hospital's real customer is the doctor," may be less true in the era of managed care. The health care center's real customers are now third–party payers, "shopping" plan members, and beneficiaries.

Don't be afraid. Tell physicians when their expectations are outdated. Tell them why their assumptions are wrong. Insist that physicians accept and meet their responsibilities. A majority of physicians will respect that approach and support you.

Mistake 4—Expecting "Loyalty."

Many executives believe they can buy a physician's loyalty. But organizational loyalty may not be part of a physician's experience. As one physician said, "If the hospital wants loyalty, let it buy a cocker spaniel." See Chapter 8 for further discussion of the "loyalty" issue.

Mistake 5—Thinking that educating and involving physicians is a waste of time.

The executive's world is a complicated mix of financial intricacy, political maneuvering, legally related activities, satisfying requirements of external agencies, and external relationships with other organizations. Some executives consider developing the support of physicians an unwelcome intrusion on their time. But many other executives have discovered that time spent developing the support of reasonable physicians is productive time indeed.

Mistake 6—Being perceived as unavailable.

When one physician calls another, the call is put right through. When a physician calls an executive, he or she is told that the executive is in a meeting and cannot be disturbed.

Of course, a totally "open door" policy is a mistake. The executive staff cannot be at the beck and call of each physician who wants to pursue a pet project. Establish and disseminate clear guidelines about availability. The best policy is probably to post a sign that says, "I'll talk to anyone about anything, but not just any time."

Mistake 7—Failing to put the monkey of adequate communication on the backs of physician leaders.

A physician executive can be particularly effective in helping physicians establish intrastaff communication. The fact that each physician wants to hear everything directly from the chief executive officer must be acknowledged, and rejected. But the executive staff can be sure that physician leaders understand the importance of, and have the skills to accomplish, timely communication between the executive/management staff and the health care center's physicians.

Mistake 8—Delegating physician matters to a junior executive or middle manager.

Think of dealing with reasonable physicians as if they are senior executives of other companies. This is usually a more productive strategy than the more natural tendency to flaunt one's authority. Senior executives of other companies would not respond favorably if told to deal with the organization through a middle manager.

Mistake 9—Believing the health care business really is identical to other businesses.

For more than a decade, *similarities* between health care services and commercial businesses have been emphasized. That parallel has proven valuable in many respects. For example, the continuous quality improvement principles of Deming,[1] and Juran,[2] and Berwick[3] are welcome additions to the quality equation in health care organizations. But "similar" and "identical" are not synonyms. Thoughtful executives now speak of *differences* between providing health care services and running a commercial business. For example, in a commercial business, the total goal is profit. Can profit be the only goal of health care centers, when a nation depends on them to provide services to people of all ages, social stations, and economic status?

The biggest difference between health care services and commercial businesses is the presence of the practicing physician, who sets systems in motion with subjective, relatively uncontrolled decisions about how to diagnose and treat each patient. As "practice guidelines" evolve, the factor of subjective practitioner behavior may diminish in importance. If and when that day comes, it will be much easier to keep health care systems well–oiled and running smoothly. But anticipating the future does not solve today's problems, many of which are related to physician factors.

Mistake 10—Being slow to establish the position of medical director/vice president of medical services.

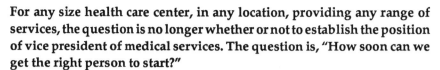

For any size health care center, in any location, providing any range of services, the question is no longer whether or not to establish the position of vice president of medical services. The question is, "How soon can we get the right person to start?"

Even if the medical staff once rejected the idea of having a vice president of medical services, the issue should be readdressed. Physicians increasingly understand the disadvantage, to physicians and those working with them, of having part–time medical staff leaders available only for breakfast, lunch, and supper meetings (also see Chapter 7).

References

1. Deming, W. *Out of the Crisis*. Cambridge, Mass.: MIT Center for Advanced Engineering Study, 1986.

2. Juran, J. *Juran on Planning for Quality*. New York, N.Y.: The Free Press, 1988.

3. Berwick, D. "Continuous Improvement as an Ideal in Health Care." *New England Journal of Medicine* 320(1):53-6, Jan. 5, 1989.

Chapter 5

Eight Common Mistakes Physicians Make

All physicians do not make the following mistakes. But these behavior patterns, even in a small number of physicians, are often significant factors in the executive–organization–physician relationship. Physician executives can be particularly effective in helping business–trained executives recognize these factors and in helping physicians avoid self–defeating attitudes and actions.

Mistake 1—Refusal to recognize a higher authority.

Remember, the physician was once Captain of the Ship. And the physician is still the "executive" in the context of treating or operating on an individual patient. That is, the activities of health care center employees involved in direct patient care, and the variable costs of patient care, are largely determined by physicians' judgments, reflected in prescriptions and "orders." Plus, systems of direct patient care are still often subject to physician approval or veto. For example, policies and procedures needed as part of infection control may be subject to medical executive committee approval.

Thus, it is hard for physicians to understand that, in terms of organizational structure, they are responsible to a higher authority, the governing body. It is even harder for physicians to swallow the fact that decisions and actions of the senior executive staff carry the weight of governing body authority.

The idea that someone might have authority over a physician is a concept that still eludes many physicians.

Thanks to the efforts of physician leaders and executives, physicians increasingly understand that acting as if they are in charge, when they really are not in charge, is a counterproductive and self–defeating strategy.

Mistake 2—Overgeneralizing

Some physicians are among the best at making snap judgments, jumping to conclusions, and overgeneralizing. And it is a matter of fact that some physicians have encountered executives who have a secretive, manipulative style. In addition, it must be acknowledged that some executives rather enjoy the reversal of roles in hospitals. That is, the "superintendent," who had to check every move with physicians is now the organization's chief executive, entrusted with board authority. Beyond that, some physicians have even heard executives state, in the context of setting up an adequate medical staff office, "That's an awful lot of money to spend on a non–revenue–producing department." So some physicians seem almost eager to believe the worst about health care executives.

Conscious effort by the health care executive (even the physician executive) is required to demonstrate personal characteristics of competence and trustworthiness.

Mistake 3—Refusal to take time to understand and use key principles, such as organizational skills, and how "the law" works.

Executives take reasonable advantage of organizational skills, such as delegating tasks. Physicians active in the organization, but primarily clinicians (such as clinical department chairs), often do not learn, or trust, organizational processes. For example, one department chairman objected to a bylaws provision stating that "department chairs provide for weekly continuing education opportunities," on the basis that he "does not have time to prepare that many conferences." Even more common is the still-existing notion that physicians must write their own bylaws! Of course, staff leaders make some decisions, such as the degree of organizational complexity, but language (word choices) in medical staff bylaws should *not* be those of a staff member "interested in bylaws."

Equally harmful to physicians is refusal to learn, or accept, how "the law" works. A good executive urges compliance with relevant statutes, attention to "process," and awareness of relevant judicial precedents. But physicians may think these matters are a waste of time. (Note that this tendency relates to refusal to accept a higher authority.)

Some physicians (don't overgeneralize) adopt a stance that conveys the **message, "I disagree with this regulation and the need for that procedural step; therefore I will proceed in my own way and, of course, expect to prevail." If not corrected, such a stance can create jeopardy for both physicians and the health care center.**

The following is an excerpt from a letter to the author, written by a physician member of a medical staff reorganization task force:

Dear Dr. Thompson,

Thank you for taking time to respond to my critique of the third draft. I am persuaded by most of your comments, and I have told Dr. (Chief of Staff) so. But I would say that I philosophically disagree with you that we should adopt the attitude, approaches, and tactics of attorneys. I am well aware that they seem to be winning every encounter with us, but history never remembers those who collaborate or capitulate in a positive light.

The writer of the letter is responding to the suggestion that, like attorneys, physicians should choose words carefully, specifically define terms, validate assumptions, and ensure fairness. Physician executives are often the key catalyst in helping such physicians understand that attention to such matters does not make them Quislings.

Mistake 4—Believing that only practicing physicians understand the details of medical practice.

In a pending malpractice case, one issue crucial to both the physician and the health care center is disagreement between a physician and an experienced nurse about a specific point in the care of a patient. A physician witness for the defense has stated, on the record, that any board–certified physician can be assumed to use judgment superior to that of any registered nurse. That assumption (already costly to the patient and family) may turn out to be costly to the involved physician and to the health care center in which the unfortunate occurrence took place.

Lots of people besides physicians now understand details of clinical care. One organizational application of this fact is to consider whether the analyst of physician performance data must always be a physician.

Mistake 5—The "George Steinbrenner Mistake." (Things not going well? Fire the manager).

Seasoned executives make necessary decisions, take necessary actions, and keep updated resumes in their desk drawers. One never knows when a rump group of unhappy physicians might urge the board to "fire the manager" (in this case the senior executive staff), assuming that a change in executives will bring back the good old days.

This problem may be lessening, as more physicians understand that the vacated position will only be filled by someone who must make the same or similar decisions, if the health care center is to be successful in the competitive marketplace.

Mistake 6—Overresistance to change.

Questioning change is not bad. Is the change really progress, or is it change for change's sake? But the Gloria Patri mentality ("As it was in the beginning, it is now and ever shall be...") is a mistake. Holding on to obsolete notions makes one vulnerable by continuing behavior that once may have been protective but isn't anymore. The only constant in the world is change. Those who wish things to remain at all the same must accept the need to move with the times. This fact is as painful for executives as it is for physicians.

 Some wise executives generate physician support by stating to physicians that health care executives are also uncomfortable with, threatened by, and fearful of changes in the health care system.

Mistake 7—Thinking that the general public still loves and has confidence in the medical profession.

Patients and family members are usually happy with their own physician. On the other hand, newspaper "Letters to the Editor" and legislative initiatives urged by interest groups indicate that "the public" believes "the medical profession" and "hospitals" have become uncaring and make too much money.

As one physician said, "Once, we were on a pedestal. Now, I don't think we are anywhere near the museum."

This public attitude toward doctors (and toward health care centers that advertise and flaunt the profit motive) may be justified to some extent. But it is also a reflection of today's society. Trust in government and big business has become a national joke. "Whom can you trust," someone might ask, "except savings and loan associations, politicians safeguarding public contributions to the Social Security fund, and Pete Rose?"

In such a society, saying, "I'm a doctor, trust me," doesn't work any more. Physicians must be helped to understand that it is to the benefit of physicians, as well as of health care centers to provide information confirming effective performance. And it is good to choose words carefully when expressing one's views. During the 1988 Presidential campaign, the head of a "Doctors Against Dukakis" group was asked why these doctors were against Dukakis. "Because," replied the physician, "Dukakis appears to be pro–patient."

Mistake 8—Being arrogant.

Review this chapter.

Chapter 6

Eleven Keys to Establishing the Executive–Physician Relationship

The following eleven suggestions reflect two basic guidelines for executives (including physician executives) and two basic guidelines for practicing physicians. The two basic guidelines for executives are:

- A condescending attitude toward physicians, hoping to win support by catering to all expressed wants and needs, is not a winning strategy. Rather, help physicians understand "the givens" in today's health care environment, how to help themselves by accepting responsibility for themselves, and how to participate effectively in today's complex health care organizations and care delivery models.

- The goal is not a short–term, limited, opportunistic relationship with a few physicians, such as in joint ventures or purchasing physician's practices. The goal is a long–range, mutually beneficial working relationship, characterized by trust.

For physicians, the two basic guidelines are:

- Cooperation with reasonable, honest health care executives is not "collaboration with the enemy." Mutually beneficial postures need not be incompatible with either the noble goals of the medical profession or the physician's economic goals.

- In an organization, the principle of ownership prevails. In the context of caring for an individual patient, or in the doctor's own office, there may be no higher authority than the doctor. But in organizational matters, the highest authority is the governing body, which expects the senior executive staff to exercise that authority in day–to–day decisions and actions.

Suggestion 1—Take the initiative.

Because of past conflicts and misunderstandings, neither traditional–thinking physicians nor traditional–thinking executives can be depended on, in every situation, to take the first step toward each other. Physician executives are ideally suited to initiating, or improving, communication and cooperative efforts.

 Look for opportunities to seek, and gain, participation of reasonable physicians in activities of the organization.

Suggestion 2—Help physicians understand "the givens."

Clear the air. Provide physicians with opportunities to understand the realities of today's health care environment. Bring in speakers, or take physicians to relevant conferences, so that physicians hear unpleasant facts from someone in addition to local executives.

Suggestion 3—Reestablish Square One.

 This year's response may be more positive than last year's. Don't let past events cloud today's decisions.

This means avoiding the assumption that it's no use discussing a given issue with physicians, because "you know how they reacted when we brought it up a year ago." Go ahead, reintroduce the issue. The reaction might be different now, especially if executives have recently been effective in helping physicians understand "the givens." Or if a vice president for medical services is now part of the picture to act as an effective liaison. Or if the executive staff has learned to explain the issue better, in terms understandable to physicians.

Reestablishing Square One also means acknowledging past events and past perceptions of each other, including mistakes and careless actions that may have resulted in wounded egos. Pursue each issue on its merits, as uncontaminated as possible by emotional reactions to previous events.

Suggestion 5—Help people hear each other correctly.

This is a true incident. An executive new to the health care field asked at ◀ ◀ ◀ a meeting, "Where is Dr. Jones?" A physician replied, "He's closing," meaning that Dr. Jones, a surgeon, was in the operating room finishing an operation. "That right?" said the new exec. "I didn't even know he was planning to sell his house."

Television sit–coms are usually based on situations created by misunderstanding, misinterpretation, miscommunication, and malassigned motives. Some interactions between physicians and executives sound like situation comedies.

"Income from operations" means one thing to the executive staff, something else to a surgeon. Then there was the time the marketing department tried to explain epidemiologic data to a physician group. Referring to a decreased mortality rate, the presenter stated, "So you can see that people aren't dying as much as they used to." One physician's prompt response was, "My patients are."

Many times, miscommunication between the executive staff and physicians is not funny at all, and can create serious problems. A current example is efforts of reasonable executives *and physician leaders* to include efficient practice habits (meaning, "Consider the patient first, but be alert for instances in which ordered services do not really contribute to the desired patient result") in physician performance reports (meaning, "If you are made aware that ordered services are really of no benefit to the patient and may indeed cause the patient discomfort, perhaps cost and quality can be served simultaneously").

Some physicians create an "us vs. them" environment by referring to such efforts as unfair "economic credentialing" (meaning an effort on the part of "administration" to abuse the physician reappointment process by limiting or revoking a physician's privileges solely on the basis of information about the cost of caring for that physician's patients, sometimes because "administration" wants to "get rid" of the physician in question and cannot prove "poor quality").

Accurate communication is not all that is needed, of course. There are real differences to be resolved and substantive issues to be negotiated. But isn't that all the more reason to be sure executives and physicians hear each other correctly?

Suggestion 6—Don't overexplain.

Remember the child who asked, "Where did I come from?" After the father uncomfortably explained reproductive processes, he asked, "What made you ask me that?" "Well," said the child, "Johnny says he came from Boston, so I just wondered where I came from."

When diagnosis–related groups (DRGs) were introduced in the early 1980s as the basis of paying hospitals for acute care services, hospital executives were, of course, anxious that physicians understand the impact of physicians' "orders" on hospital finances. Some of them initially asked physicians to listen to descriptions of complicated payment formulas, presented by the hospital's chief financial officer. Some physicians did not even sit through these explanations; others made it clear that they didn't see any reason to change their practice habits. Physicians proved to be more cooperative when the facts were made clearer, in simple language. For example, "If you were having your house painted, would you rather contract with the painter by the job or by the hour? The answer is by the job, of course. Because then time overruns, spilled paint, and cost of supplies are the financial responsibility of the painter, not the payer.

"Well, doctor, for Medicare and Medicaid patients, the government has been contracting with hospitals by the hour, so to speak. Reimbursement was an appropriate term, because there was at least a relationship between the amount the hospital was paid and the cost of treating each patient.

"Now the contract is 'by the job,' so that your hospital stands to lose money because there will no longer be a relationship between the actual cost of treating the patient and the arbitrarily established standard amount paid to the hospital under DRGs. 'Reimbursement' is no longer an appropriate term, because the amount paid to the hospital is fixed by diagnosis, and is unrelated to patient–specific differences in necessary care."

The point is, physicians did not need to become familiar with the details of complicated payment formulas. They needed to understand the relationship between hospital payment and subjective clinical decisions. (A side point is that executives did not further the image of trust when physicians in some settings were urged to design patient treatment plans and complete patient records in the manner that would put hospital payment concerns ahead of patient care concerns.)

A danger here is the narrow line between simple, effective explanation and coming across as condescending, without much confidence in a physician's ability to understand complicated issues. Keep it simple, but don't be condescending. Again, notice the value of having a physician executive, with combined business and clinical expertise, design and present effective explanations to the staff.

Suggestion 7—Demonstrate that "quality" is truly a high organizational priority.

Some physicians, and others, use "quality" as an argument when pursuing self–serving goals. But, remember, don't over–generalize. A majority of reasonable physicians truly want health care executives to be concerned about patients and family members.

Physicians will be observing total quality management (TQM) efforts very carefully. Will they see that quality initiatives relate to questions of dependable performance from the standpoint of patients and family members? Or will they be turned off by examples of the effectiveness of TQM that relate to goals of the health care center and its management? (One early example is a proud report that TQM has resulted in a reduction in the amount of lost revenue that occurred because of miscommunication between the pharmacy and patient billing).

If the executive staff considers physician support and loyalty important, they will provide substantive evidence that quality really is Job One.

Suggestion 8—Help physicians appreciate the importance, to physicians, of selecting effective physician leaders.

Physician executives can't do it all. Other key physician leaders are still often selected by the physicians themselves. For many years, physicians have been urged to appreciate the importance to *the health care center* of selecting effective leaders. Now, help physicians understand the importance *to physicians* of selecting leaders with (or who are willing to develop) organizational skills and a reputation for objectivity and fairness. For example, an important role of a clinical department chair is to be the major catalyst for communication between organizational executives and managers and practicing physicians.

Suggestion 9—Both physicians and executives should acknowledge the roots of their behavior.

Many physicians are frustrated and frightened because expectations of unlimited income and exalted position are being disappointed. Don't be afraid to tell physicians that executives feel the same pressures. For example, executive training is build, build, build. Now, in a contracting economy, the steady dependable executive who can *maintain* an organization is most valuable. That isn't as much fun, and the goal of maintaining an organization instead of building a bigger one is not even acceptable to some traditionalist executives.

 Individuals and groups who learn to discuss common concerns often discover areas in which mutually beneficial, cooperative efforts can be pursued.

Incidentally, one root of negative behavior toward physician executives, if it occurs, may be resentment that the unique cross–training of these individuals makes them a sought–after commodity in an uncertain economic environment for both physicians and executives.

Suggestion 10—Genuinely seek physician input, listen to it, and respond to it.

More than one physician, over the years, has complained, "Administration gets us together saying they want our input, but then they lecture to us about what they've already decided to do."

Listen to practicing physicians. Take suggestions when they are helpful and reasonable. But be equally comfortable clarifying to a practitioner that responding to a suggestion doesn't mean that you have to take it. Responding may be a matter of explaining to the physician that the suggestion cannot be taken because it is impractical or is based on a self–serving analysis of the situation.

Suggestion 11—Don't be arrogant.

 Interactive skills ("people skills") are as important as data, financial, and planning skills when success of plans depends in part on the cooperation of others. It is particularly difficult for people with power to accept the need to relate to others. The executive and the physician are both powerful people. So it's understandable that building the relationship is so difficult and requires such conscious effort.

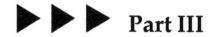 **Part III**

Some Practical Examples

These examples are merely for demonstration to focus thinking and start discussion. Of course, strategies that fit exact situations must be designed and implemented.

The author is not an attorney and does not represent himself as such. Comments and suggestions in this book are not legal advice and must not be construed or relied on as such.

Chapter 7

Developing the Position of Vice President for Medical Services

Developing the Position

(Note to reader: If the position of vice president for medical services is already well–established, skip to "Relationship with the CEO," page 42.)

The question is no longer whether to have a vice president for medical services. The question is, "How soon can we get the right person to start?" Advantages of the position of vice president for medical services include at least:

- Fills a major gap in the organizational structure by guiding and supplementing efforts of part–time physician leaders, essentially establishing a chief operating officer for medical affairs. This is an advantage for medical staff members, as well as to the hospital.

- Relieves other executives of physician–related duties.

- Provides an effective advocate to deal with external licensing and accrediting agencies.

- Provides a valuable communication link at the "chief executive officer/board/medical staff leadership/medical staff followship" interface. Because of this function, the vice president for medical services should not be viewed as "just another vice president" to be selected by the CEO without MEC and board input, solely on the basis of criteria used in hiring and firing other executive staff whose duties involve only business expertise and satisfying only the CEO.

- Provides readily available access to responsible physicians, such as by nurses and other direct patient care personnel, in the context of current patient care, total quality management, utilization management, and risk management.

- Provides an effective interpreter to help physicians understand executive decisions and why they are necessary.

- Provides critically important help to medical staff leaders and the CEO in dealing with questions of physician performance, disregard for rules, disruptive behavior, suspected impairment, or unethical practices (although the primary purpose of this position is *not* to be a "medical corrector").

Disadvantages of establishing the position of medical director/vice president for medical services are primarily transitional. For example:

- The position does not fit well into the traditional medical staff structure, in which the executive function is entrusted to a committee. (But the position does fit the modern medical staff structure, which must be part of a total quality management system (see Chapter 13).

- This position doesn't fit well into traditional executive/management structure, either. For example, the CEO may (justifiably) feel that the selection, evaluation, and firing of other senior executives is strictly up to the CEO. But if the CEO takes a dictatorial approach to filling the vice president for medical services position, refuses to accept that the position has "dotted line" accountability to the medical executive committee as well as a "solid line" reporting relationship to the CEO, or views this person as a "token physician" instead of a qualified executive with an MD or DO degree, the results of establishing the position will likely be disappointing.

- Funds must be appropriated to create this position.

- Selecting the wrong person can result in disaster. A vice president for medical services who considers him– or herself responsible only to the medical staff (a "separatist" orientation) may not fulfill responsibilities to the health center. On the other hand, a vice president for medical services who views him– or herself as just another vice president, without a unique relationship to the physician staff, may generate opposition from physicians.

- When the position is first created, fear and distrust may not be limited to physicians. Patient statesmanship with executive staff, other personnel, board members, *and* physicians is more important than any fast-track moves.

As can be seen, none of these "disadvantages" should dissuade anyone from establishing this position. Items on this list are really examples of why tact and diplomacy must be high on the list of candidate characteristics. Other desirable characteristics include unfailing integrity, persuasive communication skills (without being secretively manipulative), knowledge about current trends in health care delivery systems, and a sense of humor. In addition, the vice president for medical services must be an excellent analyst of causative factors in conflict situations and an accurate judge of people. The ability to forge acceptable compromises (in every good sense of the word) is a distinguishing characteristic of the successful vice president for medical services.

There are two kinds of people in the world: position–takers and problem-solvers. The vice president for medical services must be a problem-solver. Taking sides on even one issue can destroy the effectiveness of the position, as well as the credibility of the individual currently holding the position.

Another desirable characteristic is a thick skin. The ability to accept and respond to criticism gracefully is important. And the vice president for medical services must remain calm and even–tempered when others try to provoke a quarrel.

Some individuals, including activist physicians, control meetings with a skillful blend of provocation, intimidation, and distraction. The combination of analytical skills and thick skin enables the vice president for medical services to avoid such traps.

One commonly asked question is, "Should the vice president for medical services have a clinical practice?" Once, the answer was, "Yes, because it will increase this individual's credibility with physicians." Now, the answer is, "No, because this is a full–time job (to say the least); physicians must understand that this individual is being selected to exercise organizational skills, not clinical skills; and it is not necessary to continue practice if the individual already understands the realities and problems of clinical practitioners."

More important in gaining physician support is the "critical event." That is, the new vice president for medical services, alert for such an opportunity, solves a thorny problem or relieves unwelcome pressure.

Example: The new vice president for medical services had been introduced, individually, to many staff physicians. Some received him politely, two or three with disparaging remarks, and the majority with a "wait and see" attitude. At the quarterly staff meeting, the staff president presented a new policy tightening requirements for completion of patient records. One of the staff's bombastic orators took stage to explain that this was another ploy of administration to discredit physicians, because suspensions for failure to complete medical records were now, of course, reportable to the National Practitioner Data Bank. The vice president for medical services clarified, from a valid source, that suspensions reported to the National Practitioner Data Bank are only those related to questions of physician competence. "Administrative" suspensions, such as for failing to complete patient records, need not be reported.

Following the meeting, two or three staff members came up to the vice president for medical services with additional questions. Over the next few weeks, the vice president for medical services, careful to work with elected medical staff officers and department chairs, came to be viewed as a valuable resource by many influential members of the medical staff. (Simultaneously, the influence of the bombastic orator was seen to decline.)

Relationship with the Chief Executive Officer

The vice president for medical services must, of course, report directly to the chief executive officer or to the executive vice president, depending on the size and structure of the senior executive staff. But the working relationship between the CEO and the vice president for medical services is not totally defined by a solid–line reporting relationship. The exact nature of this relationship must be carefully decided, with relevant input from the governing body chair, the medical executive committee, and executive staff whose assignments may change. Then, all physicians, board members, executive and management staff, and relevant health care center personnel must be carefully oriented to the exact level of authority that the vice president for medical services is being allowed to assume.

The role of the vice president for medical services varies from one organization to the next. A position description must be carefully framed. Specify responsibilities related to executive/management staff activities, governing board activities, medical staff leadership activities, and community related activities.

The vice president for medical services should initiate a frank discussion with the CEO about job description *and* between–the–lines expectations. Not all CEOs expect the same thing of a vice president for medical services. Each of the following scenarios has been observed. Which do you think are appropriate, and which are not?

CEO A, president of a 500–bed medical center with a variety of inpatient and outpatient health care services, basically wants a token physician. This CEO considers having to deal with physicians as "hand–holding" and a great waste of time. He would rather pursue contracts, acquisitions, political action, and other activities related to his idea of "the health care business." This CEO seeks to pacify physicians by creating the position of "medical director," with a lot of visibility but very little authority. In fact, the vice president for medical services may be disappointed to discover that some meetings of the senior executive team take place without him or her.

CEO B, in a similar setting, views the position in terms of economic goals. He or she wants an entrepreneurial individual eager to establish new revenue–producing medical services. This vice president for medical services will be fired if he does not soon generate revenue far in excess of his annual salary, perks, and office support.

CEO C is primarily concerned with vulnerability created by lackadaisical physician leadership. For example, the health care center faces a focused survey by the Joint Commission on Accreditation of Healthcare Organizations because of "deficiencies" in "medical staff functions." And, in a just–settled case, the plaintiff's attorney came dangerously close to exposing recredentialing procedures as pro forma. Finally, in another legal near–miss, a physician was denied clinical privileges for good reasons, but almost prevailed because physician leaders ignored rules of procedure that they felt "took too much time." So, this CEO wants the vice president for medical services to work with administration, with medical staff leaders, and with the governing body to establish better medical staff/board functions as part of the health care center's total quality management program.

CEO D (the one with whom every vice president for medical services should want to work) understands that a physician executive need not be unidimensional. This CEO expects to have a close relationship with a vice president for medical services who can help planners know whether their financial projections are reasonable, given the vagaries of physician behavior and expenditures necessary to provide a quality product to the community. At the same time, this CEO believes that the vice president for medical services should be interested in helping physician leaders develop organizational skills. And this CEO expects the vice president for medical services to be genuinely interested in providing leadership to the total quality management process. Finally, and perhaps above all, this CEO actively demonstrates that the vice president for medical services is no token physician, but a valued member of the senior executive staff.

 The CEO's words and actions carry the weight of governing body authority. The CEO must make it clear to physicians and others that words and actions of the vice president for medical services carry the weight of governing body and CEO authority.

A productive working relationship between the chief executive and the vice president for medical services includes at least:

- The vice president for medical services reports directly to the CEO (or Executive Vice President in a multilayered structure).

- Meetings of the senior executive staff always include the vice president for medical services.

- The vice president for medical services is an ex-officio member of the governing body, with or without vote. (It is assumed, of course, that the CEO is also a board member).

- The CEO and the vice president for medical services attend conferences and seminars together and discuss their interpretation of information presented.

- The CEO and the vice president for medical services discuss their disagreements in private, presenting a united front to the executive/management staff, the board, and medical staff leaders and followers.

- The CEO and nursing leadership have the right to expect that the vice president for medical services will deal promptly with important patient care matters, working with attending and consulting physicians and medical staff leaders.

- The CEO expects the vice president for medical services to assume responsibility for the medical staff office. This means good management skills, such as budgeting and selecting and supervising qualified personnel.

- The CEO is entitled to expect the vice president for medical services to stay updated on physician–related requirements, such as of state agencies and the Joint Commission on Accreditation of Healthcare Organizations, and to help lead the effort to achieve compliance.

- The CEO does *not* want the vice president for medical services to play lawyer. The health care center's attorney can provide legal advice. On the other hand, the CEO must have confidence that the vice president for medical services is conversant with legal issues related to credentialing, confidentiality, ethical life support, and other matters of mutual importance to the executive staff, the medical staff, and the board.

- The CEO expects the vice president for medical services to help medical staff leaders present short, simple reports at meetings of the governing body or of relevant governing body committees.

- The CEO accepts reasonable suggestions from the vice president for medical services, related to effectively dealing with physicians.

The vice president for medical services is entitled to expect the CEO to recognize his or her unique combination of executive skills, medical knowledge, and interpersonal skills.

The CEO is entitled to expect that the vice president for medical services will sometimes cause fellow executives to forget that this executive is an MD or a DO and will, at other times, cause physicians to forget that this MD/DO is an executive.

Chapter 8

The Issue of Physician "Loyalty"

"Physician loyalty" must not be a euphemism for barely legal tying ◀◀◀
arrangements between health care centers and physicians.

Now, more than ever, health care centers are forced to compete for physicians. In some hospitals/medical centers, this effort is assigned to the marketing department. There could be no greater argument in favor of establishing the position of vice president for medical services. A physician executive is infinitely more qualified and better prepared to understand the probable reaction of different types of physicians when "loyalty" to the organization is the central issue.

Also, the vice president for medical services seems best positioned to remind the chief executive officer and the board to keep sight of the legal, and moral, duty to "exercise reasonable care in the selection of a medical staff and in granting specialized privileges,"[1] including selecting practitioners who are "worthy in character and matters of professional ethics."[2]

By 2001, the question of physician loyalty should be resolved. Physicians and health care centers will be intimately related through some version of managed care plans, effective regionalization, and capitation payment. However, predicting the future does not resolve today's dilemma. The executive staff, the governing board, and physician leaders must cultivate physician loyalty, while at the same time avoiding a hornet's nest of possible problems. For a moment, don't even think about possible antitrust problems, such as with joint ventures designed to tie physicians and their patients to the health care center. And forget, for a moment, that ignoring Medicare fraud and abuse statutes and "safe harbor regulations" could lead to fines or prison terms. Rather, step back and consider the physician loyalty question from a broader perspective, including an expanded 1990s notion of "quality" and "medical ethics."

A commonly asked question is, "To attract and keep loyal physicians, should we buy physician's practices, offer practice perks, or both?" But will long-range goals be met by throwing money at physicians? Or, as so often happens, will conventional wisdom turn out to be folly? Can loyalty really be bought? Or might one who will "sell" his or her loyalty sell it again when a higher bidder comes along? It's true that spending money is necessary to develop a nucleus of loyal physicians. But there's a big difference between attempting to buy the physician's loyalty directly, as opposed to investing wisely in efforts designed to *win* the physician's loyalty.

The ethical consideration comes in when one starts to consider the professionalism, dependability, and integrity of a medical staff built with this strategy. Will the best qualified and most committed physicians really be attracted? In addition, think of the message being sent to the nucleus of careful and caring physicians currently on the medical staff. That clear message is, "We overgeneralize about physicians to the point of thinking that all physicians are greedy and arrogant." One who might think "Well, not too far wrong," should think through the medical staff roster again. Think, perhaps, of the characteristics of physicians chosen to care for one's self and family. The point is that many physicians, contrary to public opinion it seems, preserve values of professionalism and dependability. It would be a mistake for the health care center to lose the respect of these individuals.

Next, shouldn't one carefully consider more than legal and economic aspects of joint ventures with physicians? A joint venture is an excellent idea if it makes business sense. Perhaps the joint venture is in a focused clinical area, such as an MRI Unit with radiologists.[3] Or perhaps the availability of joint venture capital makes it possible to provide a medical service previously lacking in the community. Or perhaps costly duplication of services can be avoided.

But joint ventures entered into for the expressed purpose of tying physicians and their patients to the hospital may run afoul of more than legal traps related to antitrust and other relevant legal issues. What about the impact of such ventures on clinical decisions? Surely every physician, except a superhuman moralist, might be influenced to order a certain diagnostic test, or admit the patient to one hospital instead of another, if increased income is a factor. Care must be taken that a specific joint venture is not fee–splitting raised to a sophisticated level.

There is another commonly asked and troubling question. It's usually asked by a member of the governing board. "When physicians admit patients, they use our equipment, and we pay for it. They use our nurses, and we pay the nurses' salaries. So, physicians just *owe* the health care center their loyalty, don't they?"

Theoretically, yes, in the best of all possible worlds. And some physicians see this altruistic point. But, usually, as in any human relationship, the physician's loyalty must be earned and deserved.

What should be done, then?

Let's take a fresh look at the physician loyalty question, starting at square one. What is it we expect of the physician? What does it mean to be "loyal"? According to *Funk and Wagnall's New Standard Dictionary*, loyalty = devotion = a strong attachment or affection expressing itself in earnest service.

Affection? Emotional attachment? These are unrealistic expectations. Better to remember the physician who said, "If the hospital wants loyalty, tell 'em to buy a cocker spaniel." John Gardner points out that, "The loyalty of the professional man is to his profession and not to the organization that may house him at any given moment."[4] A few physicians, mostly in the general community hospital tradition, really love their hospitals. But hardly any physician anywhere feels affection for today's multilayered "health care organization."

But is it reasonable to focus on "devotion and earnest service" as reasonable goals. These can be earned, in any relationship, by:

- Demonstrating interest in the other's ability to achieve reasonable goals, instead of always demanding that the other (person or organization) show interest in one's own goals.

- Being up front and honest with each other.

- Developing loyalty through a track record of actual decisions and actions, as opposed to lip service and promises left unfulfilled.

This perspective suggests a five–point plan:

1. **Ask the physicians!** How can you help, from their perspective? Of course, beware of some physicians' notion of "input," which is, "If you ask my advice, I expect you to take it!" And be careful to sift the wheat from the chaff. Clarify to physicians that not all ideas can be implemented. And when you judge a suggestion impractical, don't just ignore it. Prepare and give an explanation of why the suggestion cannot be implemented. Believe it or not, reasonable physicians will accept a well–documented, logical explanation and will make their next suggestions more practical.

2. **Evaluate the services you presently offer physicians, and consider new ones.** Conventional wisdom says a physician referral service is a big help to your medical staff. Is it, or isn't it? Ask. Meanwhile, offer new services. How can you help the physician with office paperwork? Do you provide a "beeper" service and computer time, free? Some hospitals provide a convenient means for physicians to dispose of harmful waste products from their offices. Conduct "personnel skills" seminars. Most physicians can't hire, fire, establish salary scales, and evaluate employees very well. Some say physician loyalty will be won by those health care centers that best help physicians organize and run outpatient practices.

3. **Don't overlook or abandon traditional physician concerns.** Most physicians still talk about being attracted to a medical center by good nursing, readily available subspecialty consultation, and a medical staff office that is more than just leftover space from marketing and risk management.

   But a caveat: Requests for expensive equipment are, of course, traditional. Here, being up front and honest pays off. While a physician's idea of "adequate equipment" may be too rich for the blood of today's budget–conscious health care center, that may be obvious only to the board and the executive staff. Have enough confidence in your reasonable physicians to share honest financial performance figures and projections with them. Plus, be honest with yourself. You *don't* have enough money to fill each physician's toy box. You may gain respect (and loyalty) by explaining that you will not be exploited; gaining physician loyalty does not mean you should be expected to play Santa Claus.

4. **See that loyal physicians have the biggest say in the organized medical staff.** Membership and political privileges are still as important to many physicians as clinical privileges. Be sure the medical staff bylaws give membership privileges (voting, holding office, being selected department

chairman, influencing operating suite and intensive care policies, etc.) to staff members who frequently bring patients to this hospital.

5. **Finally, or perhaps first of all, ask physicians, "How are we doing?"** That is, in the eyes of reasonable staff members, are the executive staff, governing board, and physician leaders earning physician loyalty by being straight and up front? Are negative 'surprises' being avoided? Do grassroots physicians feel that requested input is considered? When the CEO or vice president for medical services tells the staff something is going to happen, does it really happen?

Deliver on promises, and avoid the mistake of thinking secrets can be kept from the medical staff. Otherwise, efforts to develop physician loyalty, however heavily funded and in spite of short–term success, will probably fail in the long run.

Don't try to develop physician loyalty and generate a direct profit at the same time. To make money, the health care center must spend money on high–quality services, employee benefits, *and* some services to the health care center's physicians.

Finally, if considering a joint venture with physicians, think of the following:

- Are there other sources of investment capital that should be considered, because the motivation of tying the physician's practice to the health care center may be a questionable reason for entering ventures with physicians?

- What will be the effect of the venture on the health care center's relationship with needed physicians who do not choose to be part of the joint venture?

- Don't do a joint venture because it seems to be the rage. Is this a service that the community and its people really need?

- Don't throw the term "joint venture" around too loosely. Help physicians understand the difference (profit–loss sharing, tax advantages, etc.) between a partnership, a corporation, and a joint venture.

- Keep in mind that the executive's driving motivation is likely to be profit and tax advantage, plus control; the physician's driving motivation is likely to be control, plus profit and tax advantage. (Remember, don't overgeneralize.)

References

1. *Johnson vs. Misericordia Community Hospital.* 301 N.W. 2nd 156, Supreme Court, Wisconsin, 1981.

2. *Minimum Standard for Hospitals.* Chicago, Ill.: American College of Surgeons, 1919.

3. Thompson, R. "Trustee Melds Technology Goals of Compensating Hospitals." *Trustee* 38(12):27-30, Dec. 1985.

4. John Gardner, quoted in Toffler, A. *Future Shock*, New York, N.Y.: Random House, 1970, p. 146.

Chapter 9

Relieving Physicians' Confusion About Quality Initiatives

Executives, physicians, and others remain confused about quality ◄◄◄
initiatives. Here's why, and how the physician executive can clarify the
quality issue for all concerned.

Are continuous quality improvement (CQI) and total quality management
(TQM) synonymous? What's the relationship of CQI and TQM to traditional
QA (Quality Assurance)? What *is* "quality," anyway?

Stating specific "quality questions," each associated with a matching "quality
initiative," can clarify the total quality picture. This approach is more
productive than debating which is the entire elephant, the trunk or the tail.
Five quality questions can be stated and defined.

**Quality Question 1—Do current medical practices make a difference in
terms of altering disease processes and affecting patient outcomes?**

In the 18th Century, accepted practice was to drain blood from patients by
leeching and phlebotomy, thus removing "bad humors." What currently
accepted practices may someday appear equally primitive and erroneous?
And if two treatments are equally effective and safe, but one is much more
costly, why not take advantage of this knowledge to use the less expensive
alternative?

Some are surprised that such a body of information does not already exist,
but it does not. One reason might be opposition to such research by
practitioner interest groups fearful of the results. For example, what if it

were shown that physical therapy and manipulation were as effective as riskier, more costly surgery for many people with back pain and related symptoms?

The quality initiative related to Quality Question #1 is efficacy/effectiveness research."[1] Academically designed clinical research studies must determine, over time, the impact, or lack of impact, of a given treatment choice on the course and outcome of a patient's illness or injury.

Effectiveness/efficacy research studies might be done by individual academic medical centers, but nationwide (perhaps worldwide) pooling of information is a necessary part of this effort. This research effort need not be a quality initiative in most health care organizations, except to provide needed data to research centers. The federal government is pursuing such studies, with an interest in eventually controlling health care costs as well as improving health care quality.

The movement to establish "practice guidelines" also relates to Quality Question 1.

Quality Question 2—Are provider units (practitioners plus the health care organization) carefully applying currently acceptable diagnostic and treatment modalities?

Quality Question 2 is one of aggregate performance, like the won–lost record of a baseball team. The matching quality initiative focuses on data about what happens to groups of patients, with several factors, such as patient mix, severity of illness, etc., carefully built into the data system. Interpretation of these data must include conclusions about the degree to which:

- Aggregate institutional performance is centered on the needs and concerns of patients/family members.

- Information confirming acceptable aggregate performance is developed and shared with the public.

- Information from patient/family encounters is used to continuously maintain and improve aggregate performance.

Example: The (properly adjusted) rate of life–threatening anesthetic complications (overall or for certain procedures) in Hospital A is 7 percent, while in Hospital B it is 21 percent.

Again, note the political and legal sensitivity of quality data. Hospital B can, of course, be expected to favor keeping this fact confidential. The irony is that hospital A may also want to keep these data confidential, fearing interpretation of any clinical data by attorneys or by untrained individuals, including the press.

Addressing Quality Question 2 is not totally a matter of interpreting data. Another useful activity is reviewing current policies and procedures. What is stated in management policies, compared to the governing body's noble mission statement and the organization's corporate culture guidelines? Are specific patient care procedures appropriate when viewed from the perspective of patients, and are they effectively followed by all personnel involved in direct contact with patients and family members?

With respect to the medical staff, what is the medical staff's policy (bylaws provision, rule, or regulation) regarding needed coverage of the emergency department? Does this policy reflect the social contract implied when one chooses to be a physician?

Quality Question 3—Is each practitioner, employee, manager, executive, and board member performing dependably?

As with a baseball team, theatrical production, or any other "team" endeavor, aggregate health care results are the sum total of individual efforts.

In baseball, the won–lost record of a team (aggregate outcome information) **cannot be used to evaluate the performance of individual players. Individual statistics must also be kept, such as batting average and error rate (fielding percentage). Similarly, in health care, it should not be assumed that information related to Quality Question 2 can somehow be used to answer Quality Question 3.**

The matching quality initiative is developing, interpreting, and using data about individual performance. Conclusions about these data must include the degree to which:

- Individual performance matches clearly expressed expectations to which the individual is adequately oriented.

- Information from patient/family encounters is used to continuously maintain and improve individual performance.

- Information confirming acceptable individual performance is developed and shared with the public.

The idea of developing physician–specific performance data still troubles many physicians. Traditional "peer review" stopped short of this necessary end–point, except for flagrant instances requiring "corrective action" of a legalistic and punitive nature. This negative tradition has conditioned physicians to fear all physician–specific information. Ironically, this fear has delayed accumulation of positive information confirming *dependable* physician performance.[2]

Physician judgments set health care systems in motion, influence quality, and also determine variable (patient–specific) costs. Using the acute care setting as an example, the decision to "admit" a sick or injured person is traditionally a physician decision. Hospital personnel and equipment are placed at the physician's disposal. Through an "order sheet" in the patient's record, the responsible physician determines the activities of employees such as nurses, of diagnostic departments such as radiology and imaging, and of treatment areas such as the operating suite. The responsible physician also judges when the patient has achieved maximum benefit of treatment and so may be "discharged" from care.

 A "total quality management" system is not truly "total" unless objective conclusions about physician performance are trended and periodically communicated to each physician, as well as to individuals and groups responsible for physician performance.

One of the biggest challenges in the quality field is replacing case–by–case, negatively oriented, "peer review" methods with methods of tracking physician performance over time, including the accumulation of positive data confirming dependable performance.

Quality Question 4—Are the systems, service, and communication aspects of care contributing positively to the needs of patients, family members, and each worker in the health care workplace?

Systems and communications are important in health care because several people of varying disciplines share responsibility for the welfare of the patient. Service aspects of patient care are important because total care involves much more than careful application of clinical knowledge and skills. It is important, for example, to discover and deal with patients' and family members' feelings and fears. And it is important to realize that a "patient" is still a person who appreciates reasonable amenities.

The relevant quality initiative is application of continuous quality improvement principles in health care organizations.[3,4,5]

Conclusions must include the degree to which:

- Service to patients and family members is given high priority.

- Necessary systems function smoothly.

- Communication and cooperation between workers and the health care work place is promoted.

- Communication between "on–line" care providers (including support services such as admissions office and security) and users is accomplished.

Quality Question 5—What *is* quality?

In the academic, philosophical context, quality remains an elusive, ethereal concept that defies definition and probably always will.

The traditional assumption that quality is impossible to define is useful only in the context of quality question 5.

Pursuing the nature and spirit of quality requires the use of at least a portion of the disciplines of philosophy and ethics. It would be a human tragedy if pursuit of practical quality questions should cause abandonment of efforts to discuss, write about, study, and pursue a wide variety of concepts about the basic nature of "quality."

Here's an example of how this approach to quality helps relieve practical problems:

The Joint Commission surveyor may ask, "Are you trending outcome data?" The answer should be "Yes."

"Then," the Joint Commission surveyor might say, "give me an example."

"Certainly. The adjusted anesthetic complication rate (overall, for certain procedures, or by physician) in the first period is 4 percent. In the second period, it is 6 percent. The important conclusions are the range is 4 to 6 percent, the average is 5 percent, the increase is not statistically significant, and in both periods, the anesthetic complication rate is both within national norms and below our 'threshold' of 10 percent."

"Now show me," says the Joint Commission surveyor, "how you use that information in the reappointment of anesthesiologists."

Note the transition from Quality Question 2 to Quality Question 3. That is, statistical interpretation of aggregate data does not provide specific information about which complications were related to physician performance and which were not. So trended conclusions about the performance of an individual anesthesiologist are not available for use at reappointment time. This medical center may get a Type I recommendation from JCAHO for inadequate use of quality information in the process of reappointing individual physicians.

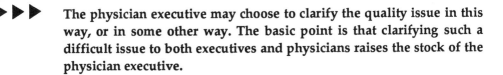 **The physician executive may choose to clarify the quality issue in this way, or in some other way. The basic point is that clarifying such a difficult issue to both executives and physicians raises the stock of the physician executive.**

References

1. Lohr, K. (editor). *Effectiveness Initiative: Setting Priorities for Clinical Conditions.* Washington, D.C.: Institute of Medicine, 1989.

2. Thompson, R. *Next Steps in Implementing Quality Improvement.* Wheaton, Ill.: Senss, Inc., 1989.

3. Deming, W. *Out of the Crisis.* Cambridge, Mass.: MIT Center for Advanced Engineering Study, 1986.

4. Juran, J. *Juran on Planning for Quality.* New York, N.Y.: The Free Press, 1988.

5. Berwick, D. "Continuous Improvement as an Ideal in Health Care." *New England Journal of Medicine* 320(1):53-6, Jan. 5, 1989.

Chapter 10

The Hospital/Medical Center and the Large Multispecialty Clinic

A few years ago, young physicians entering practice chose between "solo" practice and partnership with two or three other physicians practicing the same specialty. A few large multispecialty clinics, like the Mayo Clinic in Rochester, Minn., and the Ochsner Clinic in New Orleans, La., also existed, but this form of practice was unusual.

Today, a young physician entering practice may be courted by any number of large, strong multispecialty clinics, owned and governed by clinic members (physicians), and managed by an executive director. Ordinarily, the private clinic coexists, and competes, with other practicing physicians (solo practitioners or small specialist groups) in the community. Clinic physicians usually are located near, and almost exclusively use, one hospital or medical center.

This situation creates several special issues for the medical center. These issues must be addressed by the chief executive/vice president for medical services team (see Chapter 7). Often, dealing with these issues begins with a clarification of relative roles, responsibilities, and authority.

What is the relationship between the governing body of the medical center and the governing body of the clinic?

The principle of ownership prevails (see Chapter 3). The physicians governing the clinic make final decisions regarding clinic policies (including hiring, firing, budget, etc.). But the clinic does not dictate policy or procedure to the medical center. That is the prerogative of the medical center's governing body and executive staff. If the clinic wants to run the hospital, it must buy the hospital, and assume responsibility for its financial and quality performance, through a board and chief executive.

The ownership of a medical center determines the answer to "Who's in charge?" The answer is "the medical center's governing body, through a chief executive officer and his or her designees, such as a vice president for medical services."

Should clinic physicians have designated seats on the medical center's board?

They certainly might (check with legal counsel). And the clinic's board, or a "hospital relations committee," might include medical center board members.

What is the relationship of the medical center's chief executive (and designees, such as the vice president for medical services) to the executive director of the clinic?

Both the medical center and the clinic are well–served if these individuals have personality characteristics that allow them to communicate on important issues of mutual concern and avoid too intense an interpretation of competition. That is, pursuing mutually beneficial initiatives is preferred to the goal, on either side, of "taking over" health care in the community.

 In football, "competitive spirit" does not mean that offensive linemen should turn around and tackle their own quarterback. In fact, in any endeavor, overly intense interpretations of "competition" can be counterproductive.

What is the relationship of clinic physician leadership to positions of leadership (chief of staff, department chairman) at the medical center?

For purposes of this discussion, we are assuming that the medical center's medical staff includes both clinic physicians and other physicians practicing in the community. Positions such as chief of staff and chairs of clinical departments might be rotated between clinic physicians and other practitioners. Even if there is no real fear that the strong clinic group might "load" and dominate leadership of the hospital medical staff, rotation of key positions helps avoid even the perception that this might happen.

When any physician assumes a position of leadership, it is important that he or she learn to wear the right hat at the right time. For example, a clinic leader is obligated to think of the interests of the clinic and its patients. If the same physician also takes a position of hospital medical staff leadership, he or she is obligated to think of the interests of the entire community of physicians and of the medical center and its patients. The vice president for medical services at the medical center can be instrumental in helping physicians "keep their hats straight."

What safeguards are there to avoid abuses of credentialing and physician performance data at the medical center?

A medical center's credentialing mechanisms and use of specific physician performance data (formerly referred to as "peer review") must be objective, fair, and patient–protective. These mechanisms must not be used to further the interests of any physician group. Members of the clinic, and nonclinic physicians, may fear that the other group will seek to gain control of these functions and proceed to unfairly deny privileges or "trump up" accusations of poor medical care.

There are at least four levels of protection against such abuse of these patient–protective mechanisms:

1. Physician analysts of performance information can alternate between clinic and nonclinic physicians. Or, one member from each group can be appointed to work together to draw conclusions about physician performance information.

2. Oversight groups (performance awareness committee, medical executive committee) can be carefully structured to include individuals from both groups.

3. The governing body (coached by the CEO and the vice president for medical services) must be alert for attempted abuses.

4. Abuse of these mechanisms is unwise because of legal constraints, such as possible accusations of unfair anticompetitive behavior (antitrust, restraint of trade).

What is the relationship between recruiting efforts of the clinic and those of the medical center?

In one scenario, the clinic wants to add a cardiologist, but the medical center either has a nonclinic cardiology group under contract or doesn't include space, equipment, and staffing for complex cardiology services in its three–year plan.

In another scenario, nonclinic physicians want the medical center to recruit two or three family physicians to town, citing a perceived need of the community. But they also want these new physicians to be nonclinic physicians to increase referrals to nonclinic specialists. The clinic makes it known that it views such recruiting efforts as unfair competition.

There are some commonsense answers to such economic conflicts, but they often fall on deaf ears. For example, if the clinic wants a cardiology group and the medical center has one, shouldn't there at least be a trial round of discussions to see if an agreement suitable to all three parties (the clinic, the medical center, and the cardiologists) can be reached? Community surveys can shed light on whether the community really feels a need for a primary care alternative to the clinic or whether nonclinic specialists are simply trying to use the medical center to further their own interests. If the need is real, promoting competition by bringing nonclinic primary physicians to the community might be looked on favorably in the antitrust light. Antitrust laws exist to promote competition, not to protect individual competitors. So the primary care alternative might be viewed as a positive action because it creates competition. This assumes, of course, that no unfair tying agreements exist between the new physicians and either the medical center or nonclinic physicians. (The author is not an attorney; check the accuracy of these comments with legal counsel.)

Actually, there is no simple, logical, mutually acceptable resolution to many of these often–bitter conflicts. They may, in fact, be prime examples of why the competitive model in health care will eventually fail. That is, designers of the competitive model assumed that health care centers and physicians would band together to compete with other similar provider groups. Instead, health care has been characterized, since introduction of the competitive model, by bickering and greed. Thus, the real–world solution that some envision is a resurgence of planning legislation at either the federal or the state level. That is, a limit placed, by law and regulation, on the number and types of practitioners and health care centers that may exist in a given population area.

 Bickering and greed rather than mutual problem–solving efforts, invite limitation, by law and regulation, of the number and types of practitioners and health care centers allowed to exist in a given population area.

What is the relationship of the clinic and the medical center in terms of establishing a managed care plan?

The relationship, of course, should be using the strengths of the medical center/clinic combination as leverage. That is, offer third–party payers a high–quality, cost–effective provider group, whether it is called an HMO, a PPO, or an IPA. (It is not suggested that nonclinic physicians be excluded from participating in such a combined effort. High–quality physicians can be offered an opportunity to participate as active staff members, in good standing, of the medical center medical staff.)

Should the medical center show favoritism to clinic physicians or equally support development of the private practices of all physicians on the medical center medical staff?

Altruistically, the answer is clear. The medical center should support all its physicians. But, economically, this is a board policy decision that varies from one setting to the next. Before the board decides to show favoritism to the multispecialty clinic, the CEO/vice president for medical services team might remind the board to consider the following:

- Cronyism usually produces a significant number of disgruntled outsiders (see Chapter 4).

- Loyalty to the clinic may or may not be returned in kind (see Chapter 7).

- The clinic may begin to believe it can dictate policy to the medical center's board and dictate directives to the center's executive staff (essentially, take over running the hospital).

- The needs of the community may not be well–served by the medical center's decision to discourage clinic competitors.

Chapter 11

The Dilemma of Physician Recruiting

The CEO and the vice president for medical services know that:

- Increasing, or even maintaining, market share depends on forward–looking action.

- In spite of managed care plans, physicians can still influence the flow of patients to competing health care centers in a given area.

A profile of the current medical staff indicates an average age of 57. A growing number of physicians plan early retirement because of expressed frustration with "the government, insurance companies, and the lawyers." Finally, market share studies indicate that patients referred away because they needed subspecialty services not available locally are not returning.

Recruiting new physicians in several specialties and subspecialties appears to be a natural solution to these problems. Without the unique factor of "medical staff reaction," the recruitment plan could simply be mandated by the executive staff and board and pursued by marketing and planning. But the success of the plan may depend on acknowledging, and dealing with, a basic dilemma:

- On the one hand, the health care center wants to increase revenue and sees recruitment of additional physicians as a critical component of a successful strategy.

- On the other hand, physicians want more patients and more revenue, and see *fewer* physicians as a critical strategy. "As everyone knows," more than one physician may be happy to explain, "this city gets more doctors when we see the need for a partner and go get one."

The physician recruiting issue can create vulnerability for executives who assume that such attitudes are extinct. At best, the executive staff is vulnerable to accusations of invading traditional prerogatives; at worst, to accusations of unfair competition.

As with other issues, keys to resolution are a combination of traditional wisdom plus innovative approaches. Here are five guidelines:

1. Be sure board members have been adequately briefed and that they enthusiastically support the recruiting plan. Obtain a board resolution to that effect and a board directive to proceed.

2. Be up front with physicians early. Some counsel the opposite approach. That is, go around physicians, attempting to present them with a fait accompli. Theoretically, this allows plans to move ahead rapidly without risking physician interference. In actuality, the result is often backlash, delay, and a climate of distrust affecting future issues.

    N.B. "Be up front" does not mean put the issue on the table for a vote. It simply means advising physicians that a board directive has been given to the executive staff, giving the nature of the directive, and that reasonable suggestions about how the directive should be implemented are welcome. (Don't overexplain; see Chapter 6.)

3. Avoid the common error of quoting epidemiologic and market share studies. Some physicians seem to welcome the opportunity to scoff at the notion that this community needs "11.4" surgeons and "2.3" family physicians per some thousand population. Use such guidelines for planning purposes, if you find them helpful, but deemphasize them in talking with physicians.

    Rather, talk about impacts. Ask relevant questions, and evaluate the answers. For example, "If more family physicians and internists are not needed in the community, why are people complaining that they must wait three weeks to see a doctor?" Physicians will know some common answers and need not be forced to state them openly. For example, one possibility is that the same physicians who fail to see the need for additional physicians are working only three and a half days a week. Answers such as, "Three weeks is not very long to wait," would be evaluated, ordinarily, as unacceptable.

    One reason for asking pointed questions is that physicians sometimes come up with factors not considered in the health care center's planning process. These new insights might mean that it is best to reconsider the recruiting plan. If reversal of declining market share is not as simple as bringing in new physicians, the best time to know that is early in the planning process.

4. Help physicians recognize situations in which they create vulnerability, for themselves as well as for everyone else, through actions mistakenly believed to be protective. With respect to opposing recruiting new physicians, ask physicians if they are aware of unanticipated consequences of "circle the wagons" strategies in other communities. That is, a damaging domino effect can begin with a diminishing physician population. As physicians retire and are not replaced, remaining physicians become overextended. Some specialties may be inadequately covered or become totally unavailable. This can result in nursing concerns and resignations, and a hospital that once enjoyed a good reputation can develop an image problem in the community. Patients, including "loyal" families, may seek care elsewhere. At some point, the board must mandate closing beds and/or discontinuing services to decrease expenses and meet the budget in the face of declining revenues. The door may thus be opened to competing health care organizations, including managed care plans. In today's economy and competitive health care environment, some institutions find it impossible to recover fully from such a damaging spiral.

Explain that you are not *predicting* such a series of events. You are simply trying to help the physicians realize that "circle the wagons" does *not* automatically result in more patients per physician for the doctors left in town.

5. Finally, through whatever means of communication is best (usually a combination of memos, meeting announcements, newsletter items, conversations, and phone calls), make it clear that the governing body believes in the "right of first refusal." That is, explain that the health care center's first approach is to help qualified and interested physicians recruit partners in needed specialty and subspecialty areas. But also clarify, without arrogance or anger, that if physicians do not take advantage of this offer, they have exercised the right of first refusal. Explain that, in that case, the executive staff and board feel entitled to expect that recruiting efforts will not be attacked as either invasive of physician prerogatives or unfair competition.

Chapter 12

The Physician Factor in Mergers and Acquisitions

The merger opportunity looked perfect. Now it is on hold.

The merger opportunity looks perfect. Marketing and planning consultants have advised that costs can be held to inflationary increases while market share is doubled, duplication is avoided, and quality of care is enhanced. Legal advisors have carefully structured the merger to be acceptable to antitrust watchdogs. The executive/management staff eagerly looks forward to establishing vertically and horizontally integrated "centers of excellence" at each of the two campuses of the new MMMC (Merged Major Medical Center).

The executive staff believes that "physician input" is adequate. After all, the planning task force has been carefully structured to include three heavy admitters from each of the two current locations. Besides, each current governing body has two physician members and the staff presidents serve ex officio.

The merger plan, of course, calls for joint clinical privileges at both locations, a single medical executive committee with equal representation from both locations, and (anticipating an influx of new physicians attracted by MMMC) establishing the position of vice president for medical services.

Governing body support is enthusiastic. The press is alerted. Only one small detail remains—obtaining the blessing of the medical executive committees at the current facilities.

Last night, the plan was presented, for the first time, to the medical executive committees in a joint meeting. Each physician received a copy of the plan in a leather portfolio, with the physician's name embossed on the cover in gold. Advantages of the merger to each and every clinical specialty were described. The role of the 12 physician members of the planning committee was emphasized. (Five of the 12 physicians interrupted the presentation to explain they had been able to attend only one meeting, because the meetings were not scheduled at convenient times.) Both chiefs of staff stated that members of the medical executive committee should have no reservations about rubber–stamping this carefully sculptured enterprise.

Following the presentations, the medical executive committees were asked to meet separately in adjoining conference rooms (with fruit, cheese, boiled shrimp, and wine available) to endorse the exciting new plan. But one medical executive committee refused to endorse the plan, by a vote of 7 to 5. The other medical executive committee could not even vote on the plan. Many physicians walked out, angry that they were not consulted earlier. A quorum challenge resulted in adjournment of the meeting.

This morning, the merger plan is on hold. Of course, the board and executive staff have the authority to proceed. But they wisely wonder about the success of the new MMMC if several of the community's key physicians express public opposition to the plan.

That scenario, a composite of actual happenings, need not have occurred. If a vice president for medical services had been a major player, he or she might have counseled:

- Do not depend on input of a few heavy admitters and physicians who happen to hold positions of leadership this year. In addition to the formal involvement of these physicians in the planning process, make all staff physicians feel involved, through memos, newsletter items, and updates at meetings of clinical departments. It isn't necessary to go into great detail, but make all physicians generally aware of what's going on. Invite reasonable suggestions (with a clarification that responding to a suggestion means either taking the suggestion *or* explaining why it is not feasible to implement the suggestion).

- On the other hand, don't make the mistake of letting the medical staff believe that merger is a medical staff decision. Do *not* ask either the medical executive committee or general staff for a vote of "approval." Whether or not to merge is a governing body decision.

• Finally, appreciate the genuine concerns (sometimes justified, sometimes not, but genuine, nonetheless) of practicing physicians. What will "joint credentialing" mean to physicians who have primarily practiced at one of these two hospitals? How will the merger affect operating room schedules and nursing personnel? If there is going to be a single organized medical staff, won't some current staff leaders be deposed? Will physician leaders be allowed input into framing the job description for, and selection of, the new vice president for medical services? Believe it or not, concerns may be as basic as, "What will happen to my parking space?" Even if one thinks that's a ridiculously minor concern, it is best to deal with it as genuine.

Chapter 13

Medical Staff Reorganization and Leadership Development

Until recently, experienced executives avoided medical staff ◀ ◀ ◀
reorganization justifiably fearing negative physician reaction. Today,
executives risk losing support of forward–looking physicians if medical
staff reorganization is *not* accomplished.

It is time to count the cost of preserving too much tradition in medical staff
structure and functions.

How much does it cost to support activities of a plethora of medical staff
committees? What is the cost, in time and money, of preparing for "focused
surveys" by the Joint Commission on Accreditation of Healthcare
Organizations, often necessary because of "deficiencies" in medical staff
functions? What might incomplete credentialing and recredentialing
practices cost, in terms of legal liability and public image?

Now, concerns of many forward–looking physicians must be added to that
list. How can progress be made when leadership decisions must run the
gauntlet of approval by a generally apathetic staff? Should medical staff
bylaws still be a lengthy document, constantly in need of revision? Isn't
there a reasonable alternative to a confusing network of medical staff
committees? Is it time to pay the chief of staff and clinical department
chairs? What is the relationship of the vice president for medical services to
the medical executive committee?

Here's an example of how a needed physician was lost because of inadequate
attention to medical staff organizational activities. Working together, hospital

and medical staff leadership successfully recruited a much needed subspecialist. A few months after the physician came to the community, he began taking his hospital practice to a competing hospital in the area. Here are excerpts from his resignation letter:

"I did not join the staff until October 1989. In January 1990, I was suspended from the staff for failing to attend half of the medical staff meetings held in 1989...."

"Letters of suspension are insulting, especially when erroneously sent, plus I notice the sign–in practice at meetings includes a designated attendee signing in for three or four absent physicians...."

"The meeting attendance requirement is useless, because most meetings are disorganized and often accomplish little...."

"I was assigned to the infections committee. The members of the committee were surprised when I showed up, because it is unusual for physician members to attend these meetings...."

"In light of your plans to recruit more physicians, I suggest that these problems should be addressed...."

"Otherwise, your nursing and other physician support is good."

The following are just a few examples of generating physician support through attention to structure and functions of the medical staff organization:

- Physicians can have a significant role in a hospitalwide total quality management system, which traditional medical staff organizational behavior does not fit. The alternative is for the governing body and executive staff to implement modern quality initiatives, including use of physician performance data, without reference to or respect for much–needed physician input.

- Needless committees can be disbanded, and necessary committees can function more efficiently.

- Negative, legalistic corrective actions can be replaced by more positive supportive guidance and "corrective adjustment."

- Physicians who wish to develop leadership skills are grateful when the health care center offers leadership orientation and update seminars.

- Many physicians appreciate improved validity and fairness when modern credentialing, performance evaluation, and recredentialing methods are implemented. As a result, "quality physicians" support these activities as useful rather than opposing them as "busywork."

- The role of the vice president for medical services can be clarified as a resource to staff leaders rather than as an attempt to replace staff leaders.

- An increasing number of physicians resent the ability of a few staff members to delay or block needed improvements by taking advantage of complicated procedural rules.

But traditional "bylaws revision" is no longer a sufficient endpoint for medical staff reorganization. Several related issues must be addressed in a worthwhile medical staff reorganization effort, beginning with clarification of the nine purposes of a medical staff organization:

- Forwarding recommendations on medical staff appointments and individual-specific clinical privileges (credentialing) to the governing body.

- Developing, interpreting, and using physician performance information.

- Forwarding recommendations about reappointment, renewal of privileges, and new clinical privileges for current staff members (recredentialing) to the governing body.

- Providing continuing medical education opportunities.

- Providing routine, and special, reports to the governing body.

- Accomplishing communication between staff physicians, the executive staff, and the governing body.

- Reasonably updating medical staff bylaws and related rules, policies, and methods manuals.

- Accomplishing "corrective adjustment," defined as personal, but official, efforts to convince a staff member that practice habits or behavior require modification.

- Recommending corrective action steps, if necessary, to the governing body.

Organizational structure must be simplified. Key organizational elements are selection and orientation of clinical department chairs and designees; reconsideration of the medical staff executive function; and support by a well–staffed medical staff office, quality improvement office, and information services.

Reconsideration of the medical executive function is an especially important, and controversial, issue. The traditional medical staff is one of few organizations entrusting the executive function to a committee rather than to an individual. At the United States Constitutional Convention in 1787, delegates were tempted to consider placing the executive function in an "executive department of three persons, drawn from different parts of the country."[1] They had just fought to relieve oppression by King George III. But in spite of fearing monarchy, convention delegates concluded that executive authority must be placed in one individual (the President). "If there should be three heads in the national executive," reasoned the delegates, "there could be neither vigor nor tranquility."[2]

Some (including some physicians) predict that physicians will someday see the value of a smaller executive group. For example, a vice president for medical services and elected staff president might work with a small "cabinet" of physicians with organizational experience. Some physicians, however, still consider such a suggestion as equivalent to "disenfranchising" grass roots staff members. The basis of this objection is often general distrust of health care executives.

Effective medical staff reorganization is more than a change in structural elements. Functional methods must also be modernized. Traditional "peer review" methods must be replaced by more objective evaluation of physician performance. And fair, consistent credentialing methods must be used to resolve "turf" problems in granting individual–specific clinical privileges. Attention to qualifications (credentialing) and performance (accumulation of performance data and recredentialing) is as important in innovative managed care settings as in traditional hospital settings.

Developing effective physician leaders is also critical. Leadership orientation and update courses/seminars can be provided to leaders soon after their selection. The primary goal of such a seminar is to acquaint organizational leaders with necessary skills, not primarily to teach health care law. Of course, physician leaders should be advised of relevant legal considerations, but not as a primary emphasis. One necessary skill is the ability to chair an efficient, productive meeting. Of equal, or greater, importance is the development of interpersonal skills. For example, physician leaders must develop the ability to deal with performance problems directly, near the time of their occurrence. This can prevent the need for so many administrative and legal remedies ("preparing charges, investigations, and hearings and appeals.")

Finally, total quality management is a good framework for relating the medical staff to the rest of the health care organization. Some medical staff bylaws, rewritten in recent years, already call for a "senior leadership council," composed of senior executives (including nursing), medical staff leaders, and relevant support personnel. The total quality management process should include refinement and further evolution of such a communication forum among senior leaders.

The question of physician support is, of course, intricately related to medical staff reorganization. On one hand, practically any reorganization plan may be opposed by some physicians, on the basis that it represents change. On the other hand, failure to accomplish medical staff reorganization may create vulnerability for the health care organization, including loss of support of needed physicians.

References

1. Van Doren, C. *The Great Rehearsal: The Story of the Making and Ratifying of the Constitution of the United States.* New York, N.Y.: Penguin Books, 1986, p. 60.

2. *Ibid.*

Chapter 14

Ten Safe Predictions About the Physician–Health Care Organization Relationship

The future holds the promise of closer working relationships. That's not a self–fulfilling prediction. Physicians, executives, and physician executives must make it happen.

1. **Mutual trust will increase.**

   This is not a suggestion that physicians and executives will suddenly, magically, see only the best in each other. But this relationship, like many others, will be helped by rediscovery of basic values that once made the United States a leader nation. Management gurus will laud mutual benefits of cooperative effort. Exploitive profit–taking will once again be an exception. The norm will be reasonable profit generated by the triad of quality product, dependable service, and reasonable price. A relationship between marketing and product design and delivery will be established. Thus overpromising in advertising, which generates lack of trust, will be minimized.

   The continuous quality improvement influence is the beginning of this attitude change in United States businesses.

2. **Physician input to governing body and executive decisions will be more effective.**

   Physicians will learn to influence organizational decisions by viewing issues in a broader context than physician self–interest. Paradoxically, physician self–interest will be well–served by this participation. The availability of a vice president for medical services is a critical key to achieving this improved physician input.

3. **Physicians will choose to be part of winning health care organizations.**

The characteristics of winning health care organizations will include:

- Frantic attempts to buy a physician's loyalty will not be pursued.

- The stranglehold of legalisms and bureaucracy will be broken through proactive thinking, as opposed to simply reacting to laws and regulations. For example, winning health care organizations will become part of the solution to, rather part of the problem with, funding indigent care. Health care centers and systems may choose to contribute a small percentage of profits to an "indigent care funding pool." The rewards will include improved public relations and effective allocation of these funds by the private sector, resulting in reduced losses from uncompensated care.

4. **Health care organizations will choose sought–after practitioners.**

Being part of a successful health care organization will increasingly become a privilege, granted to practitioners with the following characteristics and behavior:

- Carefully applies updated clinical knowledge and skills to each patient.

- Is cooperative and pleasant with fellow practitioners, health care center personnel, patients, and family members.

- Appreciates contributions of others to the care of patients for whom he or she is responsible.

- Dependably fulfills the obligations of the medical profession, including ready accessibility (or provision for readily accessible coverage) in the event of emergency.

- Completes patient records accurately, legibly, and in a timely manner.

- Practices efficiently. That is, keeps concern for desirable patient care results the number one priority, but also considers the expense of ordered tests, treatments, and health care services.

To the surprise of many physicians, selection of such physicians over those with less desirable skills or habits will not be perceived as restraint of trade, if fair procedures are established and followed. "Correctly interpreted, the antitrust laws reflect the fact that the protection of competition in a health care market does not dictate that a hospital accord privileges to every practitioner that desires to use facilities....The antitrust laws protect competition, not competitors. A hospital, therefore, is justified in according privileges in a selective manner to maintain high standards of quality and efficiency...."*

* Excerpted from a letter to the American Medical Association from the Antitrust Division of the U.S. Department of Justice, December 2, 1986.

5. **Students in health care management degree programs will be taught how to work with physicians, nurses, and other health care professionals.**

Students will be made aware that the success of a health care organization depends, in large part, on activities of health care practitioners. Students will learn contrasting characteristics of management–trained individuals and clinically trained individuals (see Chapter 1). Unfortunately, there is little evidence of any corollary effort to acquaint medical students and residents–in–training with organizational principles.

6. **More chief executive officers will be physicians and nurses with executive training and experience.**

Individuals with combined clinical and organizational backgrounds will increasingly be in demand for top–level executive positions. These individuals will compete with individuals from other tracks, such as a chief finance officer who develops a broad perspective, clinical awareness, and good interpersonal skills.

7. **Successful physicians will broaden their notion of "patient care."**

A successful physician will do more than just order drugs and perform invasive diagnostic procedures and surgery. Broader aspects of health care problems will be appreciated and addressed. Physicians will participate in the "wellness" movement through public education and motivation.

Physicians will rediscover the social contract implied when one chooses to enter the medical profession. This rediscovery will benefit physicians, the public, and other health care providers.

8. **Health care organizations will temper competitive practices with social concern.**

The competitive model will eventually fail, because, in health care, profit cannot be the only motivating factor. One cannot always "cut the losers" when a society depends on its health care centers to provide a basic array of needed services.

9. **As patient care protocols evolve, fewer physicians will be needed.**

For years, physicians have feared the advent of "cookbook medicine." But the fact is that traditionally uncontrolled, subjective, individualized judgments of physicians can be standardized to a much greater degree than physicians care to admit. As care practices become more standardized, many activities of subspecialist technicians and nurses may not require a specific physician order. It should never be forgotten, however, that good cooks thoughtfully improve on the recipe when preparing individual dishes.

▶ ▶ ▶ **Fewer physicians will be needed. But advocates of managed care appear to agree that the factor of individualized clinical decision making may never be totally obsolete.**

10. **At the medical center of 2001, the nature of the "organized medical staff" will have changed.**

By 2001, the medical executive function will reside in a vice president for medical services, working with a small physician "cabinet," rather than in a large medical executive committee.

Medical staff bylaws, if they exist at all in 2001, will be a short, stable document, not one constantly in need of revision. Details once found in medical staff bylaws will be found in bylaws–related rules, policies, and methods manuals.

Emphasis will no longer be on organizational relations with a "medical staff" as a group. The organizational relationship will be with each physician. The relationship will depend, in large part, on the organizational role that the physician chooses to seek (see Chapter 3).

Clinical department chairmen will be selected as much for organizational skills, interpersonal skills, a reputation for objectivity and fairness, and communication skills as for clinical skills. These individuals will play important management roles (see Chapter 3). They will be paid from a "physician leadership fund," contributed to by both the organization and physicians.

Physicians will relate to executives, management, and nursing through a "senior leadership council," which may or may not still be called the "total quality management council."

By 2001, most physicians will appreciate that successful strategy is not to **battle the health care center, but to be a positive factor, without which the health care center is incomplete.**

DATE DUE

Demco, Inc. 38-293